CW00422356

BREAST HEALTH,

Dissolving Lumps

Other books by Pamela Jackson

Drowning, The Matrix of Learn Law

Synopsis: Whether we want it to or not, our thought process evolves daily, one way or another, developing new strands to the matrix of Learned Law at a high multiplying rate. This book addresses the compounding issue of this intangible and invisible matrix as we become lost within it, which can occur without notice. We don't find ourselves lost all at once. It is more like being in quick sand that is slowly sucking the individual under until they are drowning in their own learned behavior. They become so accustomed to performing or reacting in the same way, to situations they've systematically evaluated to be equal, until they can no longer perceive or feel a shift and change. This shifting or changing [in circumstances] warrants new behavior (renewed thinking). This book is a direct attack against the mental invasion of incarcerating thought patterns impairing an individual's future as well as an empowering, spirited message to every reader that they not only have the right, but the obligation, to change their mind.

Miracle or Coincidence

Synopsis: There are people who live day to day with miraculous things that happen in their lives more than once. More than once is an understatement for some. Are these occurrences a miracle or merely coincidence? This book gives a detailed account of phenomenal healings and activities experienced by the author first hand. It allows a close-up peak of the situations to grant the reader an opportunity to evaluate and analyze the events for themselves. Are people still able to perform miracles today? Are we able to be the recipient of a miracle directly from God these days? You be the judge. This book will be available as of winter 2020.

BREAST HEALTH,

Dissolving Lumps

By Pamela Jackson

ICDATT CWSM II
2019

Copyright © 2019 by Pamela Jackson

All rights reserved. This book or any portion thereof may not be reproduced or used in any manner whatsoever without the express written permission of the publisher except for the use of brief quotations in a book review or scholarly journal and individual home use of the recipe.

First Printing: 2019

ISBN 978-0-578-51782-7

ICDATT CWSM II
PO Box 46198
Kansas City, MO 64134
infoicdattcwsm@aol.com

www.icdattcwsm2.com

Dedication

For my God in this life and the life after, to my husband of 30 years and to my 11 children, I dedicate this work to you all.

With inspiration from the Holy Ghost, I followed the voice of God and assembled and tested ingredients to dissolve the lumps in my breast all for one reason. That reason was to stay healthy and live a long life because I have more desires I'm asking God to perform and one of them includes being able to leave a testimony, a legacy and an inheritance to you.

To all of my family, you will be happy for this book and troubled at the same time. This book contains an ugly secret about a common ingredient that's in several drinks and foods most of us really, really enjoy. It contributes to unhealthy breasts, but be strong. You can handle this truth and take on the challenge to look better, feel better, and be better.

With all my love!

Contents

Preface

From me to you:

It will be easy to read this book but it will be more difficult to maintain a consistent commitment to allotting time in applying this remedy. In the process of testing I learned that a modification to this application will increase collagen in the breasts, increasing the fullness and making them fluffier. It had a lasting effect but again, it took a commitment to applying the remedy nightly. You'll learn more about this as you read.

Although this remedy contains natural products that have been proven to fight or prevent cancerous cell growth in the body, no testing was performed using this remedy on anyone with cancer. If you have breast cancer, this book may or may not provide a solution for you to investigate. I did not have cancerous lumps. They were large lumps and there was scar tissue that most women develop. For me, it seemed as if the scar tissue were a disc in the background of my breast. If this is your situation, you can dissolve this type of lump and have beautiful and healthy breasts, instead of bean-bag or lumpy feeling breasts (fibrocystic).

If there is one thing that I learned which I feel is important to pass along, it's that this remedy takes time. It took at least 20 years to develop the lumps that I had and during that time I did nothing about them because no doctor ever said it was not natural to have them. But to the contrary, I'd have regular breast examinations and each doctor (male and female) said my breasts felt normal. It has taken 3 years of applying this remedy to almost completely dissolve them. Because they had just about disappeared, I slowed down in applying the remedy. Nearing total dissolution, I'd sometimes go weeks without doing anything. While the very small lumps did not increase in size, they did not go away on their own either. By now I believe you get the point I'm trying to drive home… this takes a consistent commitment to applying this remedy daily to achieve the expected result of dissolving breast lumps and developing heathier, fuller breasts.

Introduction

It was along about my 51st birthday, 2016 when I noticed some sort of small lump in my left breast… or was it? I wasn't about to go to the doctor and spend money I didn't have, just for them to tell me it's nothing to worry about. After all, I could hardly convince myself that it was actually a lump anyway.

A few months later, I could definitely tell it was a lump – still unconfirmed. Why me? I wondered. Well, one thing was for sure… I wasn't going to tell anyone until I had to. That included my husband. I didn't want anyone telling me what I ought to do about it. That would mean I'd have to be willing to discuss it like it was a normal conversation piece. Eventually I'd have to deal with the lump but for now, I can avoid the issue because my new job requires that I go to bed early and rise early. This is the perfect routine to avoid foreplay and discovery. It had become an unspoken understanding that there just simply wasn't time for it anyway.

Since I wasn't ready to openly acknowledge the lump, I decided to put more focus on my current desire to lose weight. I didn't know it then, but losing weight would play a significant role in the inability to hide the lump after a while. At the same time, the things I did to lose weight created a healthy inner body that would work in my favor to get rid of the breast lump.

FIRST THE TWISTED WEIGHT ISSUE

(THE QUEST FOR A SOLUTION)

I'd always been a small framed woman, weighing 120 pounds from age 22 to 30, and this was after having 4 children early in my life. I had always been active in basketball, tennis, cycling, and bowling as regular weekly fun. I could eat anything I wanted and never gain weight. I never even thought about whether I was thin or not because the subject never came up. I was simply unaware of my thin self until I was re-married at the age of 25. My husband was 42, muscular, and sexy with a deep and commanding (almost intoxicating) voice. After several complaints from him that my bones were pressing into him and hurting when I sit on his lap, lay in his arms, or otherwise… I decided I would gain weight. I ate as much as I could that was fattening and unhealthy for a couple of years, but nothing worked. Finally, I gave up. However, after turning 30 I noticed that I began to gain weight. It was only a little at a time, but I was so excited to be getting voluptuous hips and small juicy breast that I didn't mind gaining weight. I eventually bought new clothes just because I found the new me absolutely stunning, as did my husband.

By age 40 I found myself needing a whole new wardrobe because of weight gain and not because I desired form fitting, girly clothes. This was a bit unsettling seeing as though I previously had the same staple wardrobe since I was 25 years old, only adding a new suit every Christmas and when I was hired on a new job. The only part of my wardrobe that was a constant new purchase was shoes. I didn't have to outgrow them, I just enjoyed having a pair of shoes to match every suit and a pair of tennis shoes to match anything I put on. Although I was gaining more than a desirable amount of weight, my feet never changed shoe size, until… they did. I was not willing to scrap my shoe collection so…

I set out on a quest to eat healthy in order to lose weight. The past diet plans and fasting had yielded a little weight loss but as soon as the plan was completed, I'd gain the weight back. I always gained the weight in half the time it took to lose it. It's 2009 and I decided that I needed a better plan… my own plan. Through meticulous research on the world wide web and gathering information about healthy foods, I ran across the concept of negative fruit.

Negative fruit are those fruit that require your body to burn more calories digesting them than the amount of calories they initially provide upon consuming them. Eating negative fruit on a regular basis burns calories. The question became, how much of this fruit would I have to consume to begin seeing a difference? Well the answer is, a lot. An age-old lesson I learned and never forgot is that too much of anything is not good for you. So, in January 2010 I created a fruit medley or salad made of the following:

8 grapefruit	1 cup of unsweetened coconut
8 oranges	½ cup of raisins (or cran-raisins)
6 apples	1 pineapple

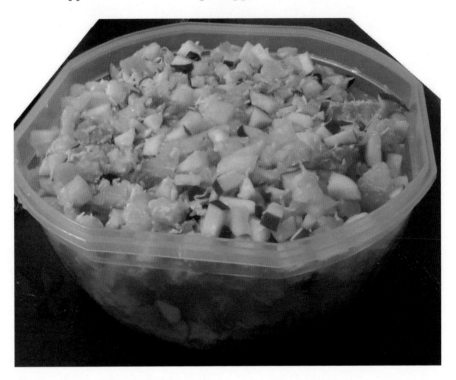

Except for the apples, I'd use a knife to cut the peel off the fruit and then cut the flesh of the fruit into pieces, discarding the core or middle. I would do this in the order they are listed above because the citrus juices from the grapefruit and oranges kept the apples from browning after cutting them into pieces with the skin on. It took a while to find the store with the best grapefruit because the flavor isn't that appealing to me. We all know that if the flavor isn't appealing, we'll likely eat much less of it, if any at all.

I felt it was time to hit the free gym offered by my employer. There was only one issue. I had fibromyalgia and although the doctor recommended plenty of exercise, it was one of the triggers that would cause muscle spasms and sometimes days off work recuperating while under the influence of muscle relaxers. Needless to say, going to the gym didn't last long. I needed pills to go to the gym and pills to recover after going to the gym. I was in a vicious cycle like so many people today. I would change medications trying to find one that was better than the other and one day I thought I'd found the miracle drug in a pill. It was caffeine. As it happened, I often got terrible headaches to the point that I needed a dark room, no noise, no smells, and the best medicine money could buy. I found that Excedrin Migraine would alleviate my headaches and blurring eyes so it became my go to medication whenever I felt a headache coming on. After a couple of years, I noticed that I had been taking fewer muscle relaxers and anti-inflammatories to relieve the fibromyalgia pain and only taking Excedrin Migraine.

During a doctor's visit in 2013 I was asked which medications I was currently taking. I said only Excedrin Migraine. They asked about the other medications, even the Allegra for my allergies and sinus headaches, and I told them Excedrin Migraine takes care of the symptoms for sinus headaches as well as muscle pain from fibromyalgia. The doctor said to be careful of taking too much Excedrin Migraine because over time it could affect my kidneys. He said it was best if I scheduled a regular appointment every so often just to keep watch on the situation. I had no problem with that, but I failed to do so. I recently had a cousin who's kidneys failed due to this reason so I'm glad the solution in the book came for me.

I was now able to do more exercise than before, but I'd learned that fat would turn into muscle from exercising and that it is more difficult to lose muscle than it is to lose the fat. Since I didn't want to 'bulk up' with muscle, I decided to slow down on the exercising until I lost weight and became slimmer.

I began eating the fruit 3 times a day in a small bowl and I ate healthy foods for two meals during the day. As I refined the menu, I began to eat meat once a day and sometimes not at all for the day. Today the meats primarily consist of turkey, chicken and fish. I eat beans on occasion and plenty of vegetables. I had to cut out salads altogether because I'd eat them dry or with a spritzer but between the acidity of the fruit and the vegetable ruffage I developed acid reflux. It was important to get that 3rd serving of fruit each night so often I'd eat it right before bed. This only aggravated the acid reflux and I'd have to lie at a tilt (bent at the waist) with my upper body propped up to relieve the chest pain from acid reflux. I experienced weight loss and then gained it again for several years before I began to learn how to be consistent and dedicated. To read about my journey go to https://weightandnutrition.webs.com. The home page has all the information you need to successfully lose weight with the fruit medley and eating healthy plan.

The victory is that I didn't give up. I began eating the fruit medley again around June 2016 and stopped during the end-of-year holiday season. It was early 2017 before I started the healthy eating plan and fruit medley again. As it did previously, the weight began to melt off each week for the first 3 weeks. During the 3rd week it slowed down but I learned that if I persevered through week 3, 4 and 5 I'd see tremendous results in week 6. During the weeks when I noticed little weight loss, I realized I was losing inches. By the time week 7 and 8 rolled around my clothes were too big and I was feeling fabulous.

This happened the first time too and I felt so great about it that I developed the website to blog my day-to-day experience. NOTE: The acid reflux didn't begin until around week 5 and I stopped the salads in week 8 and this resolved my issues after a couple of weeks. In the beginning, my husband was so impressed that he gave testimony about the effectiveness of the fruit medley to others as a conversation topic. He believed in it because he saw what it did for me. But I'd tell anyone that it takes will power and strength to stick with it. My renewed effort to lose weight again with the fruit medley was in its jumpstart phase by the time I first realized there was definitely a lump in my breast... in the middle of the year 2016. It would take almost a year before I would own it and discuss it with my husband and a couple of months after that before I talked with a physician.

My focus was healthy eating and losing weight and it took time to develop a weekly plan that worked well with other events in my life. I kept putting it off for the perfect start but then, when is it really a perfect time? I had to eventually say enough is enough to gaining weight and just get started.

Here is an outline of my weight loss journey once I had accomplished a consistent weekly plan:

1. Oct 1, 2017 ate fruit medley daily & 2 meals/day & healthy snacks
2. Splurged on outings once per week and ate less healthy meals
3. On day 14, I was 142 lbs (I started at 151)
4. 19 days after that I had consistently been 142 lbs (when I would quit)
5. I noticed I was losing inches in my waist and saddle bags (hips)
6. Nov 9th I was 140 lbs but clothes were much looser than usual
7. Nov 16th I was 138 lbs and by Nov 22nd I was 136 lbs.
8. I gained 4 lbs over Thanksgiving but by Dec 8th I was 136 lbs again.
9. On Dec 17th I was 134 lbs
10. I gained no weight over Christmas

I coasted at 131lbs from Jan thru October 2018 although I'd stopped eating the fruit medley in April. I consistently eat fruit for snacks and stick with eating mostly chicken and fish over beef and pork. I eat vegetables with most meals and limit snacking on candies, cakes and ice cream (although they are not omitted all together). Microwave popcorn is my favorite snack so I occasionally have it for my lunch and nothing else but water. When addressing your health concerns, whether it's a breast lump or something else, be sure to create a healthy inner you. You can do this by eating a fruit medley like this. As you continue to read, you'll see why this is so important.

WHY IS HEALTHY EATING RELEVANT?

Although I would eat the fruit medley for a few weeks and then quit, I knew it was the best plan for me so I kept returning to it and gaining a stronger will power each time. I've shared this weight loss journey because I believe it worked in my favor to have a healthier body while I began the effort of addressing the lump in my breast. Eating the fruit medley was primarily to lose weight but at the same time, it created a stronger immune system. I share more about this later.

I must digress back to something that occurred in 2017... By March 2017, I was the subject of a miracle, being healed of fibromyalgia... and I mean healed. I needed no medication, not even Excedrin Migraine. I write about this in my other book, Miracle or Coincidence, which is due to be released in the winter of 2021.

After stopping all medication for several months, I felt so fatigued from my work schedule and life's events that I turned back to Excedrin Migraine. It became like a daily vitamin to ward off the anticipated fatigue and keep me alert (caffeine). Just one pill a day did the trick. I could last all day, full of energy and able to stay calm under pressure. But it was after losing 20 pounds in 12 weeks and a lot of inches plus maintaining that weight loss that I could no longer hide the lump in my breast, which had enlarged. After researching breast lumps and the association of caffeine, I learned that caffeine is a contributor to breast lump growth. At this point, I'd been consuming Excedrin Migraine pills consistently since 2010 not knowing I was fueling continuous growth of a breast lump all that time.

This is an excerpt from drugs.com:

Other side effects have also been reported. In one study of the effects of caffeine, 634 women with <u>fibrocystic breast disease</u> (compared to 1066 women without the disease), the occurrence of fibrocystic breast disease was positively associated with average daily consumption of caffeine. Women who consumed 31 to 250 mg/day of caffeine were reported to have a 1.5 times increase in odds to have the disease. Women who consumed over 500 mg/day of caffeine were reported to have a 2.3 times increase in odds.

CONFESSING THE LUMP

It's all really a blur to me now but it was like an out-of-body experience. It was March 2017 and I sat on the bed and told my husband, "I have a lump in my breast". I remember silence and then talking about it. I'd lost weight in my arms, waist, sides, thighs and even my breasts. Unfortunately, the lump was increasing in size while the tissue in my breast was reduced from weight loss. The lump was very evident now and along with the lines of life (wrinkles) appearing in my breast, I felt very unappealing without clothing. That night my husband reached over to feel the lump and I cringed. I felt so abnormal. It wasn't until May that I'd find myself at the diagnostic center for a mammogram. As it happened, I made a doctor's appointment for a very general annual check-up because it was part of my insurance plan. However, I had no plans of talking about the lump yet because I just didn't feel like dealing with the prognosis.

I was visiting a different doctor this time because my doctor was retiring but as usual, the assistant asked, what medications are you currently taking? I said, for the last 18 months the only medicine I've taken is Excedrin Migraine. She said what about Naproxen, Amitriptyline, and Cyclobenzaprine? I said nope. I proceeded to tell her that I reported this information the last time I came in and the time before that but my medical record doesn't seem to get updated. I told her, I know it is hard to believe but I've had a miracle experience and I've been healed of fibromyalgia after 25 years of chronic pain. She turned toward me and looked at me very seriously with her pink and purple hair and body piercings and said, it's not hard to believe at all because God is just that good. Now, what can we do for you today?

I must say that I had probably judged a book by its cover that day because I didn't think she would relate to a miracle healing at all. My bad... I'm still learning to shed preconceived ideas learned from watching so much television in my life. The only thing I thought I knew about people that looked like punk rockers is what I'd seen on the tube... and there wasn't ever anything that had to do with Jesus and punk rockers.

I told her that I was there for the free physical and I really didn't want any charges for additional stuff. She understood and asked a couple of more times if there was anything else I wanted to discuss but I couldn't bring myself to confess. Afterward, I sat and waited for the doctor to come in. My heart warmed up to the idea that maybe the assistant, and possibly the doctor, will be understanding and gentle with my emotions and feelings if I tell them. I pondered whether I was ready to deal with this. There was a slight knock on the door and the doctor walks in announcing herself with a greeting... Hi, I'm Dr. Angel (yes, for real... that was her name)... how are we today? My answer was always the same. Well, I think I'm doing pretty good.

Dr. Angel went through all the regular probing questions as she updated my file on her tablet and then she asked if I had any other concerns. I said no and she proceeded to explain the lab work she intended to order. I re-emphasized that I only wanted what came with the free physical and we discussed insurance. She was understanding but at the same time it seemed like I shorted myself in receiving the full 'Angel Care' she would have given. On her way out, my mouth opened as if I had no control… wait, there is something else, I said. I was hesitant and she could sense my apprehension. I told her; I have a lump in my breast. She sat her tablet down and came closer to me. I wonder if she was now conflicted about giving me the 'Angel Care' or the free care.

At any rate, she asked some questions with heartwarming compassion. When did you first notice the lump? I slumped down as my head flung back and then looked at her. I lowered my eyes and said I guess it was over a year ago. I knew in my heart that any good doctor would want to chastise me for not reporting it sooner but I was comforted and somewhat stroked by her response, it's okay, I understand. Is there a history of breast cancer or lumps in your family? No, I responded. And then there were a few more questions before she said, I'm going to have someone bring you a robe and I want you to get undressed from the waist up. I'll be back to examine your breasts. After she left, I sat in the quiet room and wondered what had I just set into motion? What will she find or discover?

Quickly the assistant came back into the room with a gown and instructions. As she moved about, she asked, why didn't you tell me when we talked earlier? I said, I guess I was scared. She said there is never a reason to be scared to tell us what's going on with you. We care about you. I felt as if she was offended that I didn't trust her enough to tell her. I called out to her as her back was turned and told her that it wasn't so much as being scared to tell her, as much as it was simply not being ready to deal with it. I just wasn't ready for what I might hear. She gave a gentle smile and said, well, now we know and we'll be here for you no matter what. She touched my hand and left the room. I quickly changed my clothes and not a moment too soon, before Dr. Angel gives a quick knock on the door and announces herself. Come in, I said.

She did the breast exam with little to no discerning expressions on her face. She removed her gloves and told me I could sit up. She said the lump moves rather freely and is possibly filled with liquid much like a cyst. Do you have any pain with this? No, I said. It's not uncomfortable at all… it just feels like me. She ordered a mammogram and a sonogram so that she could be for sure but she told me that lumps form like this in many women around my age and it's not uncommon. She didn't think it was cancerous and said some women opt to have it removed if it's causing an issue. She said, if it's not causing you any pain or discomfort there's no medical reason requiring surgery to remove it. It would be your choice. It was nice of her to let me know I'm not alone but truly, in my mind it was all about me right now and not the other millions of women around my age walking around with lumpy breasts. Dr. Angel explained that after surgically removing the lump, most women experience regrowth of the lump at some point.

This is because the lump is intertwined with the normal breast tissue and when removing it, it is not possible to get the root of it. Therefore, it may be a matter of time before it returns.

I went home and shared this information with my husband and we were both relieved. Within a week or two I was at the medical center for a mammogram. I told the facilitator that the last time (and only time) I had a mammogram was over 10 years ago and it was so painful that I'd sworn I'd never do it again. I noticed that the machine looked a lot different so I asked if I could expect a different experience. She said technology has come a long way in regards to mammograms and they have a new, improved 3D machine but there is still quite a bit of discomfort when getting it done. Well, I'm here to tell you that it was no different than the first time except, instead of sucking my breast into a small wind tunnel and practically sucking it off my chest, this new machine squished it into a pancake, first top to bottom and then side to side. I know it should be my advice for every woman to get a mammogram but it's not. My advice is simply, if you choose to get a mammogram take Jesus along with you.

The sonogram was much more soothing, especially after the mammogram experience. The warm gel and massaging movement of the smooth round scanner against my breast gave me relief. When the images were reviewed by the specialist, he confirmed that I have a fibrocystic breast lump which is benign (not cancer).

NICE TEA

Since the mammogram, I've had swelling and pain in my breast. The doctor said it was normal and should go away. I think the swelling went down but the nagging soreness only around the lump was lingering for weeks and it didn't help that I had developed a very nasty chest cold. I began to pray in my mind as I moved about daily, hoping for an answer as to what to do about the breast lump. However, as my cold became worse, I laid in bed and asked God what should I do to get rid of the cold. As though it was an idea I'd never heard of, I thought ONION, get some onion and make a tea.

I know this was a message from the heavens because it came from nowhere and felt higher than my own thoughts. Such a simple thing… onions that is… but still it seemed so much higher than anything I would have thought of on my own. In just the same way, I thought of the ingredients to make a tea, which I call Nice Tea. I began researching each of the ingredients that had come to mind. I was blown away by the research. Here are some things I learned.

ONIONS

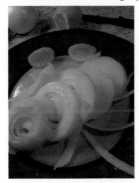

Onions have phytochemicals that seek out free radicals in your body to destroy them. These same phytochemicals reduce the risk of gastric ulcers, according to the National Onion Association. The chromium in onions help to regulate blood sugar and the sulfur aides in lowering blood sugar because it triggers an increase in natural insulin production. Onions even act as an anti-inflammatory agent. In other words, onions are useful in detoxifying the body and fighting against disease, even cancer. White onion yielded the best results for me but you can use yellow or red onions too. I experimented with all of them.

HONEY

Honey has antioxidants called phenolic compounds. Medical research suggests that phenolic compounds may have anticancer effects. Honey is heated and processed to remove impurities but during my research I found commentary that suggest honey loses health benefits when heated and may even become dangerous to your health. Sarika Rana explains in an article on the NDTV Food website, September 2017, that heating or cooking honey can cause adverse effects in the honey's composition that is not good for the body when digested, especially for those with diabetes. According to thehealthyhomeeconomist.com website, this adverse effect even applies to commercially sold honey that has been heated during the process to remove impurities. I and my husband have had no issues with consuming the cooked honey but we are pretty healthy overall. Another commentary by sleepingbearfarms.com, a honey processing company, says heating honey will not give you a horrible disease or kill you. It explains the process thoroughly and the chemical changes that take place.

Honey is added to many products you buy at the super market like barbeque sauces, beans, cookies, and more. All of these products were cooked or heated to achieve the final product with honey, not to mention the large number of recipes that call for honey during the cooking process such honey roasted 'anything', yeast rolls, pineapple upside down cake, and barbeque ribs, just to name a few. Honey provides great flavor but also helps improve cholesterol levels, improves digestion, and can kill unwanted bacteria and fungus if not heated to the point that it destroys all of its health benefits.

The average person who is healthy is unlikely to experience issues with regular consumption of honey. However, honey is high in fructose and glucose and could be harmful to people who are overweight, diabetic or otherwise required to manage their dietary intake of fructose and carbs. These people should avoid honey as well as sugars. People with health issues, especially those affected by diet, should consult their physician about using Nice Tea even though the ingredients are natural.

GINGER ROOT

Ginger root is used to fight flu and common cold and has powerful anti-inflammatory properties. Ginger root when consumed on a consistent basis helps reduce muscle pain and soreness as well as stiffness in the joints. Through testing, ginger root was instrumental in lowering risks associated with heart disease and helps to prevent the growth of abnormal cells such as those that form lumps and cancer. As a basic prevention source, ginger root simply helps to fight infection.

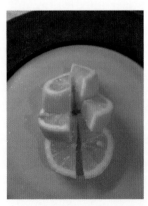

LEMON

Lemons are very high in vitamin C and according to the American Heart Association, lemons lower the risk of ischemic stroke in women (a stroke caused by a blood clot in the brain that plugs the blood vessels). Because lemons are a good source of flavonoids they help to protect against cancer and cardiovascular (heart) disease.

APPLE CIDER VINEGAR

Apple cider vinegar is made relatively the same way alcohol is made. First the sugars are fermented and turned into alcohol and then bacteria are added and allowed to further ferment, turning it into acetic acid. Vinegar in French means sour wine and thus, apple cider vinegar. Fermentation is when food is exposed to bacteria and yeasts and allowed to age (just sit). The benefit, when done correctly, is that microorganisms are created in the fermented mixture that are able to overcome and take out the kind of microorganisms that can kill us. But one thing to avoid is cooking the fermented mixture because it kills the beneficial microorganisms. The bacteria culture (bacteria, proteins and enzymes) used in the fermenting process of apple cider vinegar is called the mother. When buying apple cider vinegar for this recipe be sure to buy the kind that states 'with the mother'. Like honey, my research suggests that heating apple cider vinegar removes the valuable health benefits. However, according to Healthline.com, apple cider vinegar is used in preserving food. The process of preserving food usually involves heating the food. It is also used in creating sauces and marinades.

COMBINING THEM ALL

The benefits of the ingredients used in Nice Tea are explained in summary based on my research of existing data and studies but since I am not a medical professional, I can only apply my training as a professional analyst of 15 years. Combining these ingredients with decaf tea is the recipe that came to my mind before I ever set sail down the path of research. The research and experiments I performed was to solidify the results. Together, these ingredients shape the right internal environment to fight disease and more applicably, kill the abnormal cells that create fibrocystic lumps.

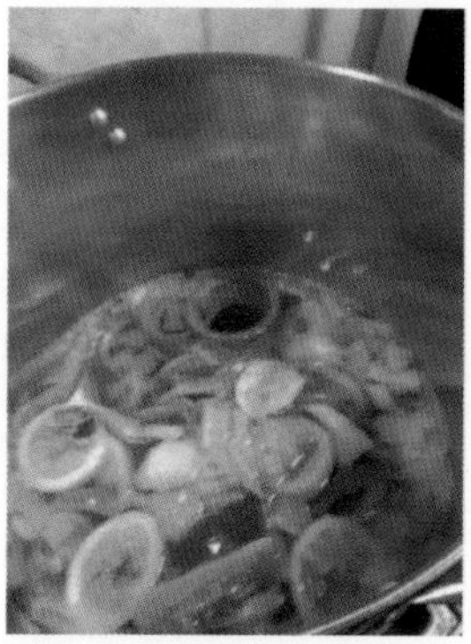

I began what I thought would be a short journey to dissolve the breast lump but it turned out to take much longer than expected. I had quick and astonishing results from the beginning but then I began to veer down the path of experimentation. I wanted to know what would happen if I changed the way I put together the ingredients and what if I only drank one cup a day or two or three? I will discuss more about the process of experimentation in the next section but the recipe I created is shown below. I call it Nice Tea.

NICE TEA
By Pamela Jackson, October 2017

4 Quarts water
1 Medium to large lemon
1 Large white onion
2 Cups of Asian Ginger tea mix
 Or substitute 1 cup of honey & ½ cup of chopped/grated ginger
½ Cup of Apple Cider vinegar (with the Mother in it)
½ Cup of Honey [NO WHITE SUGAR]
6 Tea bags (no caffeine & better if it contains rose hips and hibiscus) –
try Perfect Peach by BIGELOW and Mango Passionfruit by STASH.

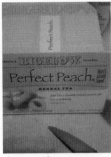
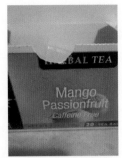

rose hips – reduces the symptoms of arthritis, lowers cholesterol and blood pressure, aids in preventing heart disease, and boost your immune system

hibiscus – provides relief from high blood pressure, lowers cholesterol, decrease symptoms of inflammatory disease. [While studies have been performed to validate this effect of hibiscus, I did not find solid scientific research referenced.]

Instructions

1.   Heat 4 quarts of water in a large pot on a high heat.

2.   Cut the lemon into pieces on a plate (leaving juice to cover the plate). You may have to squeeze some of the lemon onto the plate. Then, squeeze the juice and pulp from the cut pieces into the water. As you do this, drop the lemon peels into the water.

3.   Cut the onion into slices on the plate with the lemon juice. (the lemon juice reduces the sting to the eyes so you may want to keep a slice near the plate in case you need more lemon juice). Then break apart the sliced onion rings and add them to the lemon water along with any lemon slices you still have.

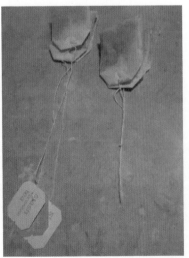

4. Add 6 tea bags (remove any paper tags). It may be best to tie a knot in the strings (tying 3 bags together) so that they do not open during the stirring and boiling process).

5. Allow the mixture to boil until the onions become thin looking. Then remove the mixture from heat and let it cool off for about 30 minutes. It should still be quite warm.

6. Pour the Asian Ginger Tea Mix into the hot tea mixture and stir (or pour in the substitute ingredients & stir).

7.   Pour in the Apple Cider vinegar and ½ cup of honey and stir. Let the mixture cool for another hour.

8.   Strain and remove the ingredients so there is only a liquid. The liquid will be slightly cloudy with fine particles from the ingredients. I found this made the tea rich and robust and was more effective. If this is not palatable for you, try straining the tea a second time with a strainer that has smaller holes. I use a strainer to remove the onions, lemons and tea bags. I squeeze them out with the back of a spoon to keep as much tea as possible. Then I use a small strainer and pour the tea from the pot into a large bowl. This requires that I rinse the strainer a few times during the process as it gets clogged with the pulp from the tea. After this, I rinse the pot and pour the tea from the bowl back into the pot again. I repeat the straining process using a second strainer with holes so tiny you can barely see them. Then I pour the final product into a pitcher. You will want to use a one-gallon sized pitcher because the recipe will yield just over 3 quarts of tea. The additional capacity in the pitcher will allow you to add more water or honey if needed to suit your taste.

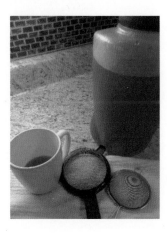 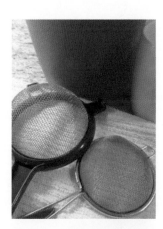

If the tea is too sweet just add a little water. Just the same, if the tea is too tart add a bit more honey while the mixture is still warm. Store in the refrigerator and drink a small tea cup amount two to three times a day to dissolve or dry-up a cyst.

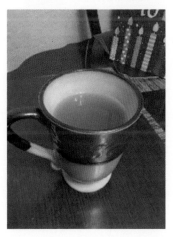

EXPERIMENTING

The recipe is down to a science for me now. I first began drinking one small cup per day and received results within the first week. After several weeks I began drinking two cups per day, once in the morning on an empty stomach and again just before bed. I would make sure it had been at least a couple of hours since I'd eaten. I also began measuring my breast lump. It was quite large and at this point, protruding beyond my skin, almost as much as my nipple.

I decided to stop drinking the tea to see if the decrease in size would continue. It continued for about a week and began to taper off. After the 2nd week there was no additional change. My husband made a comment that he could really tell the difference by touch. After several months, I could see that it was no longer protruding beyond my skin when looking in the mirror or looking down at my shirt. I stopped drinking Nice Tea again for several weeks so that I could start fresh with another experiment. When I resumed drinking Nice Tea, I decided to double the onions. However, I did not notice any increase of speed at which the lump was dissolving. To my surprise, it didn't make my breath stink either… you know, the way onions normally would if eaten raw.

As another experiment I decided to omit the Asian Ginger Tea Mix and replace it with honey and fresh ginger. I notice no difference in the effectivity of the Nice Tea. I believe this is because the active ingredient for Nice Tea is the onion. All of the other ingredients are to create a palatable tea while adding health benefits that create a healthy immune system. Toward the end of writing this book I began drinking a full tea cup of Nice Tea, three time each day and I noticed an increase of lump reduction. I would encourage you to try Nice Tea and vary the ingredients or amount you drink based on weight and height. I am 5'2 and on a good day I weigh 135lbs.

REMEMBER, the goal is to create a healthier internal body (fruit) and a stronger immune system (fruit + Nice Tea).

Nice Tea alone has added benefits such as reducing joint pain, creating fluffier and fuller breasts, aides the body in fighting against colds and flu, as well as aides in lowering high blood pressure. However, I've learned that if you aren't eating right (such as consuming lots of caffeine) you can't expect the proper results.

YOUR IMMUNE SYSTEM

In this section we'll first explore the body part that functions as our immune system (lymph nodes) and then we'll take a look at how our diet affects this part of our body.

Most people understand what veins are in our bodies. They are blood vessels that carry blood throughout our bodies. Well, there are other vessels in the body called lymphatic vessels. Blood vessels run completely throughout the body but lymphatic vessels are strategically placed in only certain areas like around and under the armpits, in the neck, in the bend of the elbows, and the center of the body and in the genital area. Although there is connectivity between the two types of vessels, in appearance they are different because the lymphatic system has small beads called lymph nodes. The lymph nodes are situated in clusters along the lymphatic vessel. The lymph nodes act as a filter for the fluid called lymph that runs through the lymphatic vessels. Another way the lymphatic vessels are different than veins is that they are closed at one end while blood vessels circulate blood from a beginning point and back to the same point and continues. In a lymphatic vessel, the fluid flows only one direction and is filtered as it moves through the lymph node clusters. Each section of lymph nodes act as a protector against germs and infection for assigned parts of the body.

To simplify the process of how the lymph fluid is created and flows through the lymphatic vessels, I will explain it without the complicated nature it involves. Nutrients and oxygen are carried through the blood vessel system from our food and other intake. The valuable portions that nourish us are carried to cells in our bodies through interstitial fluid. Most of this fluid is then returned to the blood system but about 10% of it remains behind in the tissue of our organs and body. It is a clear to yellowish liquid called lymph. The lymph will begin to flow separately from the interstitial fluid and will flow into the lymphatic vessels via the blood system. It will flow in one direction only and be filtered by the lymph nodes, after which it is dumped back into the blood system at the end of its journey.

The heart does not pump the lymph fluid through the lymphatic vessels as it does blood through the veins. Rather, the lymph fluid depends on muscles pumping properly. Breathing, pulsation within the body and the natural contraction of the filled lymph node keeps the lymph fluid moving through the vessels. In summary, the lymph nodes properly drain the fluid for each part of the body and therefore, removal of lymph nodes may prevent the fluid from being able to drain, causing the fluid to back up and create other issues. The reason I mention this is because at times it is necessary for a surgeon to remove lymph nodes when they are attached to a breast lump that has grown into the lymph nodes located near the arm pit. If surgery to remove a breast lump near the arm pit area is optional or voluntary, you should definitely consider the ramifications. Cedars Sinai is a not-for-profit hospital in Los Angeles, California. They have an educational website in which they offer a 'What It Is' page for explaining how a breast lump is removed and when necessary, how infected lymph nodes are removed. See Axillary Lymph Node Dissection in the Reference section at the end of this book.

When lymph nodes are filtering the lymph fluid, it is removing matter characterized as the enemy. That's right… it seeks out invaders like cancerous cells, infections, bacteria, and other matter that will attack our bodies, cause abnormal growths or otherwise make us sick. These invaders enter our bodies largely through what we eat. They can also enter our bodies via creams and other topical applications we use like ointments and make up. Even an encounter with nature or interaction with animals can result in unwanted germs entering your bloodstream. What we eat is super important because it is by this that we can also strengthen our immune system. We can be strategic by eating certain foods daily or throughout the week that purposely increase the health of our lymph nodes.

Consuming too much sugar at one time slows down the immune system cells that fight bacteria. So, for instance, after drinking two sugary drinks like soda or gas station cappuccinos your body will begin experiencing about 3 hours of decreased ability in cells that should be fighting against bacteria. Eating more fruits and vegetables ensure you boost your immune system with vitamins C and E as well as beta-carotene and zinc. Citrus fruit and red bell peppers are rich in vitamin C.

Let me explain more clearly how lymph nodes and eating vitamin C rich fruits and vegetables are connected. Each lymph node is surrounded by a capsule that contains collagen and lots of it. Part of the inner tissue within the lymph node is also made of collagen. This collagen is an important protein that your lymph nodes use to hold the tissue of the body together and create healthy tissue throughout the whole body. Vitamin C boosts collagen collection by the lymph node. Thus, increasing your vitamin C intake is like supplying your body's fighters with bullets for its guns. Those fighters become stronger and begin to attack invaders in the body as well as keep out additional invaders. These invaders are called free radicals and we don't want them in our bodies.

Earlier I spoke to you about how eating the fruit medley (to lose weight) would become an important part of the plan to get rid of a breast lump. I didn't know then, but I was actually preparing my immune system to attack the abnormal cells in my breast that were forming the fluid filled lump. Onions are an antioxidant, which simply means, it is a powerful weapon against free radicals in our bodies. The onion, full of vitamin C and other nutrients and vitamins, essentially help lymph nodes do their job.

SIZE DOES MATTER

Okay, now that we've dissected the solution, let's take another look at the problem. At a point of noticing a drastic change in how the lump was decreasing, I also began to notice that the measurement from one side of the lump to the other wasn't changing very much from week to week. The only reason I knew it was still shrinking is because it was sinking further into my breast, toward the center, and I could feel it less and less when lying on my stomach in bed. I could also feel strands within my breast breaking lose as if they were shrinking, then popping loose and being severed. You should be aware that this can be a bit painful at times and happens with no warning at least a few times each week. I also noticed that as I continued to drink Nice Tea, the lump was becoming very dense (or soft) as it sank into the normal breast tissue. The only way I could explain the change I was experiencing is by saying that the lump was decreasing in size on the back side.

During this new period of change, I felt another lump. I couldn't believe it. This was approximately 11 months after the mammogram. I called the diagnostic center to see if I could get a copy of the mammogram results because I began to wonder about what the original lump actually looked like. I was astonished to find out that there were originally multiple lumps in my breast and that the primary lump was not only huge, it was situated largely from my rib cage to my nipple in depth… and spread out side to side (width). The width is how I had been measuring the change in size reduction. I had no way to measure the depth so I decided I'd have to get another mammogram to truly see the change.

Here are images of the initial mammogram showing the lump. The white mass indicates fluid and not regular breast tissue. Although fibrocystic breast lumps feel solid, they are actually filled with a fluid or puss like substance and can grow to be very large, as you can see.

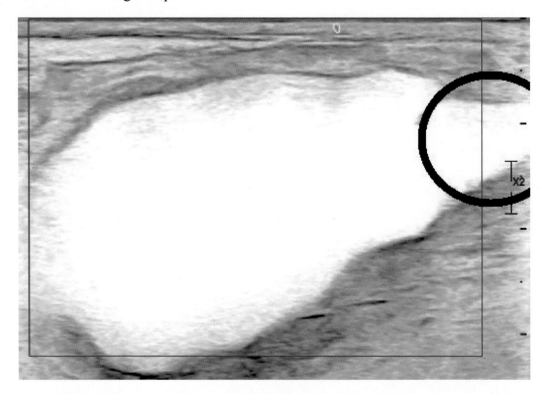

This is a side view of the lump. The part that I've circled in black is the part of the lump that is closest to the nipple, which began to protrude beyond the skin as it continued to grow. I might also mention that the lump appeared to grow faster after the mammogram than before. This could be because at the time of the mammogram, the lump was inhabiting about 59% of my breast capacity per the mammogram results. This means that as it grew it was now at the point of having very little room to expand inside the breast. Additionally, the doctor said that fibrocystic lumps often increase in size during a woman's monthly cycle due to hormonal changes. After the cycle it will go back to the way it was. My cycle had always been regularly irregular. This means that there was a pattern that could be mapped but the pattern was not monthly. It had a pattern that repeated every 3 months and then 4 months. Since I no longer menstruate it is difficult for me to track my pattern so I could not always tell when the lump was getting larger due to monthly hormonal changes.

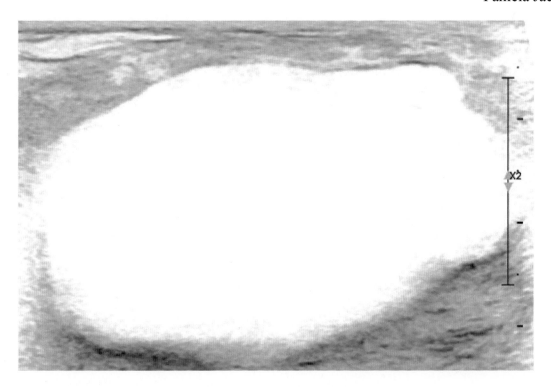

Above is a top-down view (as if I were looking down at my breast). The white portion of the circular mass is the lump. The left edge of the picture is my rib cage and the right edge cuts off just before the nipple. Below is an image that shows a bottom-up view and reveals two additional smaller lumps.

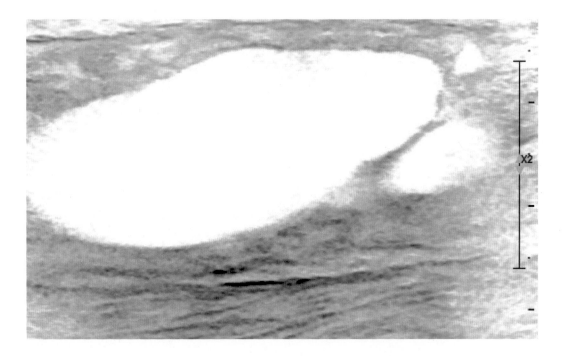

Notice the disproportioned size change when looking at the lump from the top-down versus the bottom-up. This is because the lump actually has multiple lumps fused together on top.

I made a visit to the same doctor and asked about their analysis of the mammogram. She concurred that there were multiple lumps and one primary larger one. During the examination she seemed baffled at the increased mobility of the lump. I asked her if she believed the lump was smaller and she said she really couldn't tell but it is her experience that the lumps increase in size, but don't get smaller. [I believe the lump had increased mobility because it was smaller than the first examination a year earlier.] After this, I continued drinking Nice Tea and noticed more pain as the invisible process of surgery seem to be occurring in my breast tissue. I also questioned the gristle like disc that I could feel in both my breasts. I wanted to know whether it was considered a lump also. The doctor said it was not a lump and does not appear on the mammogram as such. The gristle like matter in my breast was normal breast tissue. The doctor made another appointment for an annual mammogram but I decided not to go until months later. Now that I understood the depth of the matter (no pun intended), I wanted to give myself more time to drink Nice Tea to incur greater results.

In the meantime, I did more research as well. An article on Broadlyvice.com titled 'How Your Boobs Are Supposed to Feel' cites information derived from the Mayo Clinic. Breast tissue is made of fat, glands and support structures that include clusters called lobes. Lobes contain lobules which fill with milk when breastfeeding. These are all connected within the breast, like computer circuitry. Fibrosis is a process where the connective tissue becomes gristly. When fibrosis occurs in the breast tissue it feels the same as scar tissue, having different levels of change from a bean bag to a gristle like matter.

When fibrosis occurs in the breast it will occur in both breasts simultaneously, with the same effect. If you feel a gristle like matter or lump in one breast but don't feel the same exact thing in the other breast, this is not fibrosis normal and you should see a doctor.

Below are images of the mammogram completed after drinking Nice Tea for 15 months off and on. You'll see a significant size reduction. I've placed white nodules around the circular walls of what is now, the lump. The surrounding fuzzy looking part is the breast tissue that has occurred from fibrosis.

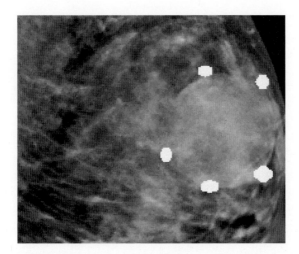

Again, the left edge of the picture is my rib cage and the lower right corner cuts off just before the nipple. You'll notice that the lump is half the size it was originally and has taken on a more definite circular shape. It now occupies about 35% of the space within my breast as opposed to 59% like before. I call this a victory for womankind.

DISCOVERY

Of course, Nice Tea is not as useful if it doesn't help other people like it is helping me so I decided to ask a few people to try my discovery. My aunt, my husband, and my daughter were among the first. My daughter couldn't get used to the flavor although she liked what she has learned about apple cider vinegar. She doesn't have a breast lump, arthritis, joint stiffness, high cholesterol or blood pressure so Nice Tea does not appeal to her as a solution she needs. She does however like to be healthy so she began adding apple cider vinegar to a glass of orange juice a couple of times per week and that seems to be beneficial for her. My aunt felt Nice Tea was helpful with joint pain due to arthritis and muscle pain, as well as high blood pressure. She began having her family drink it but she said a pitcher goes so quickly between them all that she can't keep up with making it.

My husband saw benefits of reducing his blood pressure and drank it consistently for a while. He exchanged it for beet juice to reduce his blood pressure but after several months, he decided to return to drinking Nice Tea on a consistent basis. He is experimenting with how Nice Tea affects other health concerns and maybe he'll be writing a book about his experiences one day for men who need a cure without surgery. My husband does not have cancer or any other life-threatening disease but he has other health concerns that Nice Tea may be able to address. Onions are powerful! Medicalnewstoday.com highlights a study that shows consuming more than 7 servings of onions per week was associated with a decrease in colorectal cancer. They also cited a paper published by the *Journal of the National Cancer Institute* in which a controlled case study of the effects of allium vegetables (onions) on prostate cancer revealed that men with the highest intake had the lowest risk of prostate cancer.

I went a step further to discover just what the onion can do in reducing the breast lump, and I put a slice of onion against the skin of my breast and lined my bra with a breast pad. The smell was so strong that I had to wrap myself tightly in other garments and only do this when I was at home or sleeping. I did this for 3 days on and 2 days off for about 15 days. The first 5 days motivated me to continue, even as I drank Nice Tea, because I had a decrease of aging wrinkles on my breasts. After the 3rd week I notice I was unusually lopsided one breast to the other. I asked my husband if it was just me and he said I definitely had one side larger than the other. The breast that I applied the onion to was larger and fuller... even visually with clothing on.

I began to research the effects of onions to see how this occurred. Something I overlooked by Medicalnewstoday.com is how the high level of vitamin C in onions contribute to the maintenance of collagen in our skin. I found many articles about what vegetables to eat to increase my collagen intake, which all included onions, but nothing in reference to putting onion on your skin to increase breast size. I did see astonishing results where people used fresh onion juice on their face (yikes!) and achieved tighter, smoother, unblemished skin. However, I didn't try it and can't vouch for that. What I did try, more than once, is putting onion slices on my breasts. The second time around, I did it for a week on both breasts but was not drinking Nice Tea and I had the same results, with the exception of size reduction in the lump. It WORKED! It increased the size of my breasts. The results were very appealing. I never had cleavage because my breasts weren't big enough to be that close together but I began to see cleavage after applying the onion to my skin for several weeks during the night.

If you plan to try putting a slice of onion on each breast and wrapping yourself up, here are some tips that made it work more smoothly.

1.   Use Saran wrap instead of a breast pad because it seals the juice against the skin as opposed to soaking up the onion juice into the breast pad.

2.   Only leave the onion on the skin for about 4 hours and then remove it. The onion can make your skin raw and the Saran wrap can cause the area to sweat and your skin will become temporarily discolored if left covered too long.

3.   After removing the onion, apply a thin layer of Vaseline or other protectant to the skin to keep the skin healthy.

4.   Only use it while sleeping if you won't be bothering another person in bed. The onions can be quite strong but did not burn my eyes like when I'm cutting them. It becomes a different kind of smell when you wear the onions. It is more like 'funky', really funky.

5.   Use a fresh slice of onion for each application and be consistent with 4 hours per day, 3 days in a row. Then, try to give your breasts a rest for two or three days.

I should mention that while the results this provided lasted for a long time, I don't think it is permanent. I stopped applying the onion to my skin and stopped drinking Nice Tea for about 6 weeks and during that time I slowly saw the enlarged breast begin to match the other one. I didn't incur any flatness and the wrinkles did not return but the cleavage did decrease. During this process I did not measure my breasts to see exactly how much change was occurring. I can only say that it was a remarkably visible change.

Since we're still in the discussion of 'Discovery', I should mention that I had developed a bitter/sweet relationship with the breast lump. When aroused sexually, the lump had an increased sensitivity that was pleasurable to the point that it enhanced the experience upon touch. I've become sad to see it go but NO MORE LUMPS, PLEASE.

Nice Tea has improved other health issues as well. Over the last 10 years, I've also had an increase in my rheumatoid factor. Some of my joints seem to be changing and I have fingers that are slightly turning inward. My ankles are very painful at times of walking. However, the Rheumatologist stated that my rheumatoid factor wasn't high enough to prescribe other remedies to address it. Well, Nice Tea alleviated most of the pain I was having and I actually forgot about it. That is, until I stopped drinking Nice Tea for several weeks. The joint pain returned and it seemed to take about a week of drinking Nice Tea in the mornings and at night before I experience some relief again. I still have stiffness in the mornings however, even when drinking Nice Tea.

rgg
Pamela Jackson

CONCLUSION

If you are generally healthy and have a breast lump, I recommend Nice Tea before you choose surgery. If you didn't notice, this is NOT an overnight cure. It takes time and consistency. I bought a house in July 2018 and did not have time to make Nice Tea for 5 months. It was December 2018 before I began drinking it consistently again. During that time, I had no change in the size of the lump. This is proof that it requires consistency. The good news is that it didn't get larger. I contribute this to avoiding caffeine as a regular item for consumption and eating negative calorie fruit and vegetables often each week.

You will want to pay close attention to eating healthier too. I can't guarantee results for everyone because I believe that the state of health of the individual lends to or detracts from the results each will experience. If the individual can't be disciplined enough to change their eating habits or can't change their eating habits due to medical reasons, career or other requirements then results will definitely vary.

If you have noticed wrinkles in your breasts (beyond initially waking up in the morning) or desire an increased plumpness and smoothness to your breasts, then try regularly applying onion to the skin BEFORE surgery. The only thing to sacrifice is time… it takes time to allow Nice Tea or the application of onions to work. It will also take time for you to find the right schedule and adjustments to the recipe that works for you. Currently (December 4, 2019) the lump in my breast is the size of a small marble and I've been drinking Nice Tea consistently in the morning and at night using the alternative, honey and ginger. I also drink a third cup during the middle of the day three to four times each week before lunch and I've seen better results. It has become a little smaller, and a little smaller each week. Hopefully later this year I'll have the opportunity to share results from a new mammogram with you all.

As a final thought, be sure to drink Nice Tea on an empty stomach as often as you can. I'm not sure why the results seemed better but they were. Find me on Facebook and tell the world how it worked out for you:

https://www.facebook.com/buff.author.

Inquiring minds want to know about your journey to healing or natural enhancement. If you're too embarrassed to share a personal moment like this, maybe you can ask a friend to post it for you on my Facebook page without mentioning your name. It is important to note that **THIS BOOK IS NOT INTENDED TO PREVENT OR CURE ANY DISEASE**. My only claim is to reduce the size of breast lumps and lumpiness.

As with anything, be sure to exam whether citrus (fruit, oil or juice) will affect you adversely. If you've eaten lemons, pineapples, oranges or grapefruit in the past and you've had negative results such as rashes due to sensitive skin, acid reflux or other allergies **STOP**, this solution is not for you. If you have a disease or condition, especially one that is affected by your diet, **CONSULT** your doctor first.

Oh yeah… remember to regularly examine your breasts for lumps. Monthly should be the minimum.

References

6 Proven benefits of Apple Cider Vinegar
https://www.healthline.com/nutrition/6-proven-health-benefits-of-apple-cider-vinegar

15 Evidence-based Benefits of Lemon by Kiran Patil January 3, 2019
https://www.organicfacts.net/health-benefits/fruit/health-benefits-of-lemon.html

30 Surprising Uses for Apple Cider Vinegar
https://www.healthline.com/nutrition/apple-cider-vinegar-uses

A Detailed Guide to Ginger: What's In It, Why It's Good For You and More by
Rena Goldman, Medically Reviewed by Kelly Kennedy RD
https://www.everydayhealth.com/diet-nutrition/diet/ginger-nutrition-facts-health-benefits-alternative-uses-more/

Axillary Lymph Node Dissection; Cedars Sanai Medical Center
https://www.cedars-sinai.edu/Patients/Health-Conditions/Axillary-Lymph-Node-Dissection.aspx

Does Cooking Honey Make It Toxic? by Sarah Pope MGA
https://www.thehealthyhomeeconomist.com/is-cooking-honey-unhealthy/

Excedrin Migraine Side Effects – Medically reviewed July 4, 2018
https://www.drugs.com/sfx/excedrin-migraine-side-effects.html

Health Benefits and Risks of Onions
https://www.medicalnewstoday.com/articles/276714.php

Health Benefits of Onions: 5 Surprising Ways Onions Can Cleanse Your Body to
Eliminate Disease by Lizette Borreli July 31, 2014
https://www.medicaldaily.com/health-benefits-onions-5-surprising-ways-onions-can-cleanse-your-body-eliminate-disease-295820

Health Properties of Onions, National Onion Association
https://www.onions-usa.org/media/view/14/Health-Properties-of-Onions

Heating Honey, Pros and Cons by Aaron Dexter May 16, 2017
https://www.sleepingbearfarms.com/raw-honey-posts/heating-honey-pros-cons/

Hibiscus, Web MD
https://www.webmd.com/vitamins/ai/ingredientmono-211/hibiscus

How Can My Diet Affect My Immune System? Web MD

https://www.webmd.com/cold-and-flu/qa/how-can-my-diet-affect-my-immune-system

How The Lymphatic System Works, by Jane Barton
http://manuallymphtherapy.com/manual-lymph-therapy/how-the-lymphatic-system-works/

How Your Boobs Are Supposed To Feel by Bethy Squires June 2016
https://broadly.vice.com/en_us/article/ezjjvk/how-your-boobs-are-supposed-to-feel

Lemons: Benefits, Nutrition, Tips and Risks by Megan Ware RDN LD January 2018
https://www.medicalnewstoday.com/articles/283476.php

Lymph Nodes and Cancer: What is the lymph system; American Cancer Society
https://www.cancer.org/cancer/cancer-basics/lymph-nodes-and-cancer.html

Lymph Notes
http://www.lymphnotes.com/article.php/id/151/

Reasons Why You Should Never Cook Honey by Sarika Rana September 25, 2017
https://food.ndtv.com/food-drinks/reasons-why-you-should-never-cook-honey-1696700

Rose Hip Uses and Potential Benefits
https://www.verywellhealth.com/the-benefits-of-rose-hip-89506

Rose Hip, Web MD
https://www.webmd.com/vitamins/ai/ingredientmono-839/rose-hip

Swollen Lymph Nodes; Mayo Clinic
https://www.mayoclinic.org/diseases-conditions/swollen-lymph-nodes/symptoms-causes/syc-20353902

What Are The Benefits of Vitamin C In Lymphatic Tissue; San Francisco Gate
https://healthyeating.sfgate.com/benefits-vitamin-c-lymphatic-tissue-10388.html

Printed in Great Britain
by Amazon

75547160R00029